A GUIDE FOR WOMEN HOW TO ENJOY SEX

Seven Tips That Really Work

Ashley Anne

Table of Contents

Introduction:

In spite of the fact that I've for the most part partaken in my sexual coexistence, I arrived at a point a couple of years prior where I began to ponder, "Is this it?!"

It was disappointing because I did not have any idea what I did not have the foggiest idea. How would you appreciate sex more when you do not have the foggiest idea where to begin?

I was in good company. A large number of women feel this disappointment, some for their completely sexual lives. The degree of which appears in some not exactly awesome patterns:

- Women are almost certain than men to be unsatisfied with their sexual experiences.
- Straight women have less climaxes than their male accomplices do (and less climaxes than sexually unbiased or lesbian women do).
- What's more, 10% - 40% of women experience issues arriving at climax by any means.

So on the off chance that you're feeling a bit 'meh' about sex, or you're keeping yourself up around evening time considering how to appreciate sex more, you're most certainly not the only one.

Since we are listening to this, we're not shown how to have incredible sex.

Sex in schools centers around wellbeing, contraception, and security. Moreover, keeping in mind that those things are significant, there is close to nothing about joy.

Add to this the skank disgracing and untouchable that encompasses female sexuality, in addition to the wide range of various harmful crap that stems from orientation imbalance and man centric mentalities on sex…

Overall, any reasonable person would agree that there is a great deal hindering women's pleasure.

However, the uplifting news is that you can assume control over the issues. (Furthermore, indeed, I imply that both actually and metaphorically.)

In the event that you are interested in how to appreciate sex more, these seven fundamentals will assist you with turning your pleasure dial all the way up.

They're not planned as The Total Aide for the Best Sex of Your Life. That is a profound leap of faith, a venture special to every woman, and the sort of customized work I do with my 1:1 clients.

However, on the off chance that you're bungling in obscurity pondering where to begin, these are seven strong advances you can take to appreciate sex more and make a more pleasurable, fulfilling sexual coexistence.

Give yourself an opportunity to Get Excited

Heads up: people's bodies work in an unexpected way.

Progressive, I know.

Truly, all bodies work somewhat better: what turns you on and what switches you off; how you are longing works; how you like to move in the room. We humans are complicated and multi-layered.

Yet, here is the greatest disclosure that completely shakes my reality (positively) when I first figured out how to appreciate sex more:

It's estimated that women need something like 20 minutes of sexual play to get completely stimulated.

Recently, I let that hit home: twenty entire minutes.

Actually, excitement is hard to logically study. We are sexual creatures, not machines, so times shift broadly. Moreover, keeping in mind that there is no authority agreement on what amount of time it requires for one or the other, men or women, the key focal point is this:

Sexual excitement takes time. Furthermore, it will likely take additional time than you are giving yourself.

Presently, there are really two distinct sorts of excitement: the actual excitement of your body and your abstract excitement — how stimulated you FEEL. (Moreover, negative, they do not necessarily, in all cases, cross-over).

They are both unbelievably significant for getting a charge out of sex. Moreover, keeping in mind that emotional excitement is somewhat more perplexing (favoring that in a second), giving your body sufficient opportunity to turn on is an extraordinary spot to begin.

Consider it-there a great deal of requirements to occur down there.

Additional blood needs to stream to every one of the mind-boggling pieces of your privates—enlarging the lips of your vulva, nearly multiplying the size of your clitoris, and greasing up your vaginal channel.

The sensitive spots all over your V-parts need time to initiate; turning on delight spots like your Sweet Spot, A-Spot, and that is just the beginning.

Your vagina additionally needs time to stretch. It extends up to twice its size, moving your cervix deeper into your body and farther away.

Cool, huh?

Moreover, that implies one of the brilliant principles for how to appreciate sex more is this:

Set aside some margin to fire up those motors.

Energetic kissing Bosom play fingering (with loads of regard for the clitoris). Oral sex whatever makes you happy and turns you on. In any case, in particular, give yourself way, much longer than a couple of moments to prepare for sex.

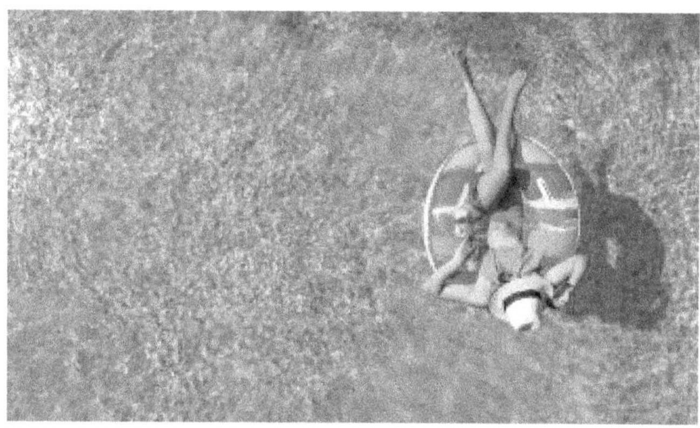

Get Your Entire Body Included

When you crack out of this world of sex, you really want something other than your privates in the game; you maintain that your entire body and mind should be stimulated as well.

We will get to the brain part in a second, but how would you increase excitement in your entire body?

You put forth the attempt to get everything required to turn everything ON:

Run your hands and fingers across your neck, your bosom, your arms, your thighs. Request that your accomplice kiss the rear of your neck and shoulders. Investigate every trace of your body, and welcome your accomplice to do likewise.

Draw in your faculties. Drink in your accomplice's body (and your own) with your eyes. Pay attention to every one of the delicious, arousing sounds. Smell the uniqueness of their skin. Get imaginative and see every one of the 'on' switches.

You can likewise use breath to move delight all through your body. Envision delight transmitting out from your privates and into every cell of your body.

You maintain that your skin should feel electric, your areolas to be turned on and hitting with delight, and your whole body to be well and really locked in.

Since regardless of your orientation, making additional opportunities for entire body excitement will assist you in getting a charge out of sex more. Every one of the faculties = all the joy.

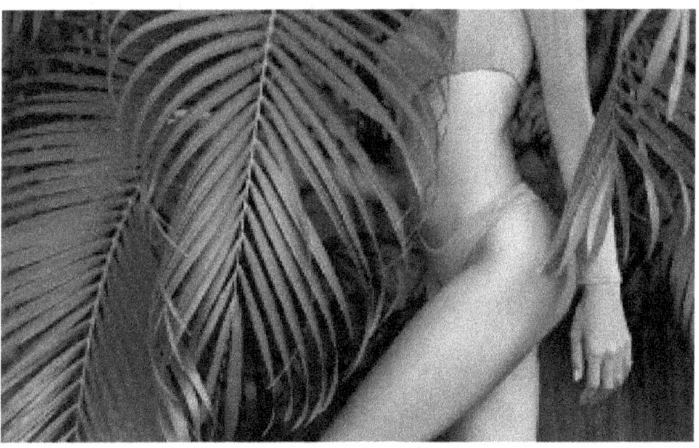

Press the Delight Button

Your clitoris is perhaps nature's most spectacular creation. With north of 8,000 hit delicate sore spots (that is the most elevated fixation anywhere in the human body-male or female), it is a super-hot joy button.

Which makes it your all in-one resource for taking a not terrible, but not great sexual coexistence to staggering remarkableness.

One of the most straightforward tips for how to appreciate sex more is to just keep your clit included. However much as could reasonably be expected Indeed, during oral sex and fingering and all of your 'foreplay' type exercises. And furthermore, during the entrance

Repeatedly, women get to the 'sex' part and disregard their clit. However, that is where the majority of the sensitive spots are—and thus where a ton of joy occurs.

Sadly, a ton of women feels shame about contacting themselves, or requiring clitoral excitement to feel joy during penetrative sex.

I get it-there's a ton of BS out there that puts vaginal climaxes on some sort of platform and causes ladies to feel 'not exactly', assuming that they've never had one.

Indeed, you can figure out how to have vaginal climaxes assuming you need to, but on the other hand, they are interesting. By far most women report requiring clitoral feeling to arrive at climax.

The lesson of the story? Offer your child a lot of consideration. Have your accomplice play with it while they are inside you. Play with it yourself. Find every one of the ways in which it gets a kick out of the chance to be animated, and track down the places that focus on you in the perfect way.

Press that delicious button, and press it frequently. That is what it is there for.

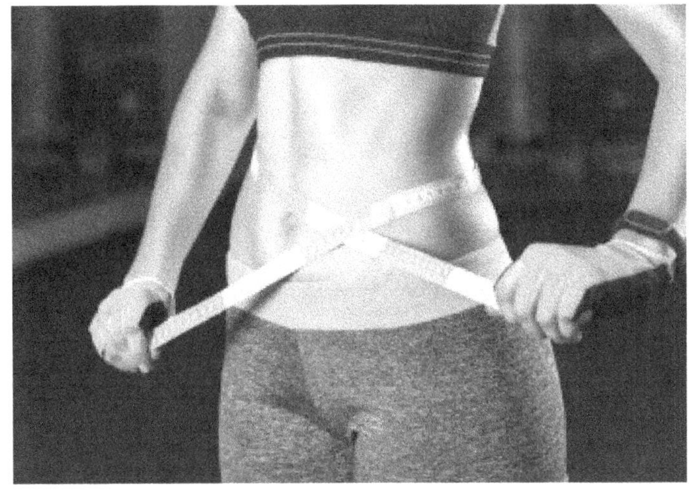

Get Your Head in the Game

We have currently covered a large part of the actual exciting stuff. Nevertheless, except if you begin doing whatever it takes to address this one, it will scarcely have an effect.

Listen to this: excitement is not simply physical- it likewise occurs in the psyche.

You can draw in your faculties and press that delight button all you like, yet in the event that your brain is not in that frame of mind, there is a cutoff to the amount you will have the option to celebrate:

Some of the time, your brain is still hustling from an insanely occupied day and an incomplete plan for the day.
Some of the time, sex is not working since there is some implicit poo going down in your relationship. (That is right, that good old glaring issue at hand will screw with your sexual coexistence more than you understand.)
In some cases, you are not having a decent outlook on yourself or your body, and sex is carrying those uncertainties to the surface.
Everything greatly affects your happiness regarding sex.

Moreover, that implies need #1 is figuring out how to unwind, having a real sense of reassurance, and feeling cherished and appreciated. Whether that is with your accomplice, inside yourself, or both,

It is more difficult than one might expect, correct?

I will not belittle you and imagine that a straightforward bullet point article has every one of the responses to the burdens and difficulties of your life. (Furthermore, we should be genuine here - hearing "simply unwind" ordinarily makes us need to punch somebody.)

Nevertheless, I will say this:

The more extensive conditions of your life have an effect on the room. You cannot carry on with an unpleasant life while hoping to have a great sexual coexistence.

Overall, resolving the more perplexing issues will have a positive effect on your sexual coexistence, and your whole life.

Simultaneously, it very well may be pretty much as basic as beginning to incorporate some unwinding time into your "foreplay" exercises:

Have a shower. Go to yoga. Pay attention to some music. Get a back rub. Work on making a space—both truly, intellectually, and inwardly—where you have a solid sense of security to give up.

By doing whatever it may take to address stressors and focus on unwinding, you allow yourself the ideal opportunity to appreciate sex more.

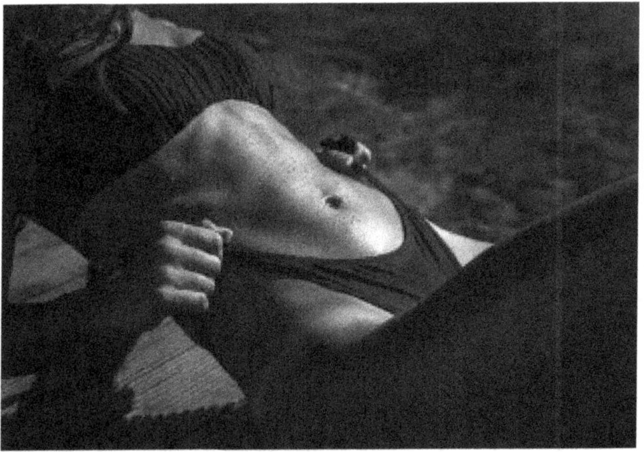

Disregard Climaxes

Climaxes are perfect. We are certainly favorable to climaxes.

Unexpectedly enough, however, you will have the option to appreciate sex more on the off chance that you quit zeroing in on it.

In the event that you are attempting to 'arrive' as fast as could really be expected (and stressing over what reason you are not), you pass up the entire experience not too far off at the time.

Therefore, here comes a possibly incredible rethink: Sex does not need to be a rush to climax. It may very well be an encounter of delight, association, and love. Then again, essentially anything that you pick it to be.

The justifications for why we have intercourse are varied and copious, and your opinion on sex has an enormous impact on your happiness regarding it.

However, a straightforward method for incorporating this will be to make an effort not to climax.

Assuming that climax is at this point not the objective, it frees you up to entire different universes of plausibility. Which thusly frees you up to more profound fulfillment and satisfaction.

At the point when you reevaluate the "objective" of sex, you eliminate the strain to climax. Which allows you to show up in an unexpected way, to partake in the wide range of various gifts of your sexual experience, and to quit agonizing over "how you're requiring."

This is a distinct advantage for men as well. At the point when the race towards climax and discharge is eliminated, it considers an alternate in-the-second insight of joy and association.

Overlooking climaxes could sound unusual from the beginning, but check it out and see where it takes you.

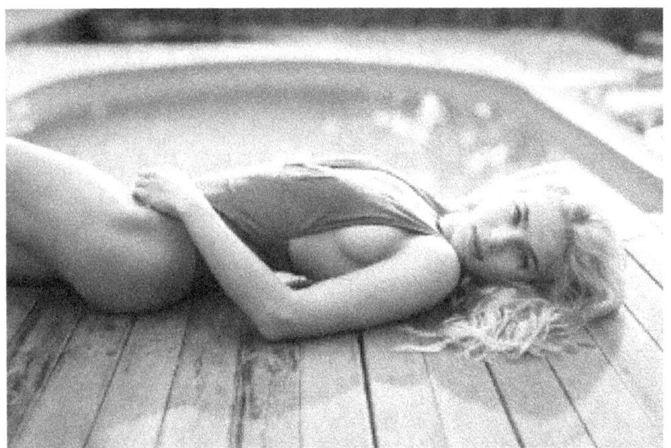

The Wetter the Better

Sex resembles a slip and slide:

Add a great deal of wetness, and you have long stretches of tricky tomfoolery. Go in dry, and you will get erosion. No, no fun by any means.

Such a large part of the disappointing women's experience during sex is because of distress.

The.

You're not loosened up adequately.

It is beginning to torment there (and not positively).

We will address the initial two in a second, yet the last one has the least demanding fix around:

Lube.

Tragically, numerous women feel humiliated or embarrassed about going after additional grease. Similarly, as men have been molded to connect the size of their private parts to their feeling of manliness, so too have women connected their womanliness to their degree of wetness.

We are calling BS.

While not being wet enough may be a sign you are not heated up yet (see point #1), requiring some additional lubrication is likewise ordinary.

Here's something clear, but not generally perceived: Ladies can be really turned on yet not exceptionally wet. What's more, we can, likewise, get wet without being turned on by any means. (Sexuality is muddled that way.)

Also, women of any age (particularly those in post-menopause) actually do not grease up a lot. Regardless of how hot and turned on they are,

So how about we ditch the disgrace and standardize the utilization of ointment (simply ensure it is the right osmolality). You can get all au-naturel and use some spit (my own number one). Then again, invest some additional energy in your number one wetness-initiating foreplay (oral sex, anybody?).

Since about getting a charge out of sex more, it is a reasonable instance of 'the wetter the better.'

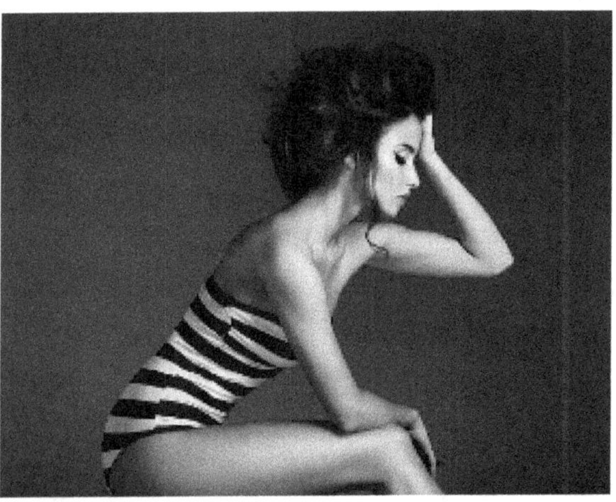

Request What You Need

Need to know one more method for tending to a great deal of sexual disappointment with one basic activity?

Request what you need.

Awkward there? Request a pad to help your legs.

That point feels a bit bizarre. Stop briefly and move around until it feels better.

Excessively hard? Excessively profound? Excessively quick? Not quickly enough?

You understand.

Requesting what you need could get a piece stopped/began off-kilter on occasion, but that is fine. In spite of what we find in the established press, sex is seldom an immaculate, impeccably executed dance. It cannot be-that is not sensible, in fact.

What IS practical is two people (or more, assuming that is the way you roll) meeting up to make a remarkable encounter.

It is acceptable for that to be a bit muddled on occasion. The fact that it is untidy now and then makes it awesome. It is the main way for it to be genuine, credible, associated, and, indeed, pleasurable.

So, to appreciate sex more, start with a discussion.

You do not need to zero in on what is going on (in spite of the fact that it has alright to voice that as well). You can approach things in a positive, development-oriented way.

"I need to hold on to developing our sexual coexistence together and appreciate sex more. Here are a few thoughts I might want to attempt..."

This can be frightening. Since voicing your longings and confronting, the chance of judgment or dismissal is defenseless,

In any case, it is this sharing of who you truly are and what you truly need that prompts further closeness. This straightforwardness at last unites you and assists you in getting a charge out of sex.

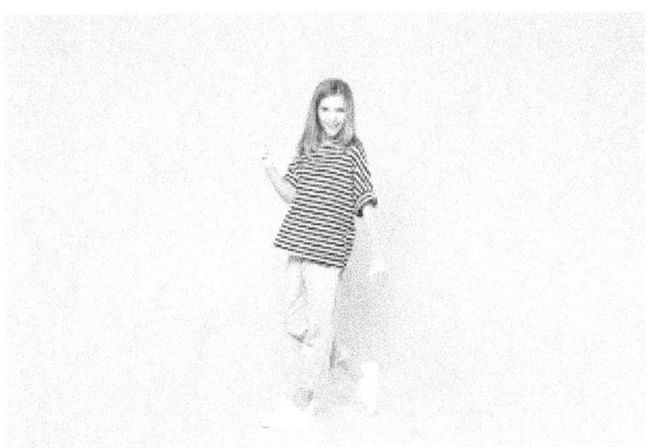

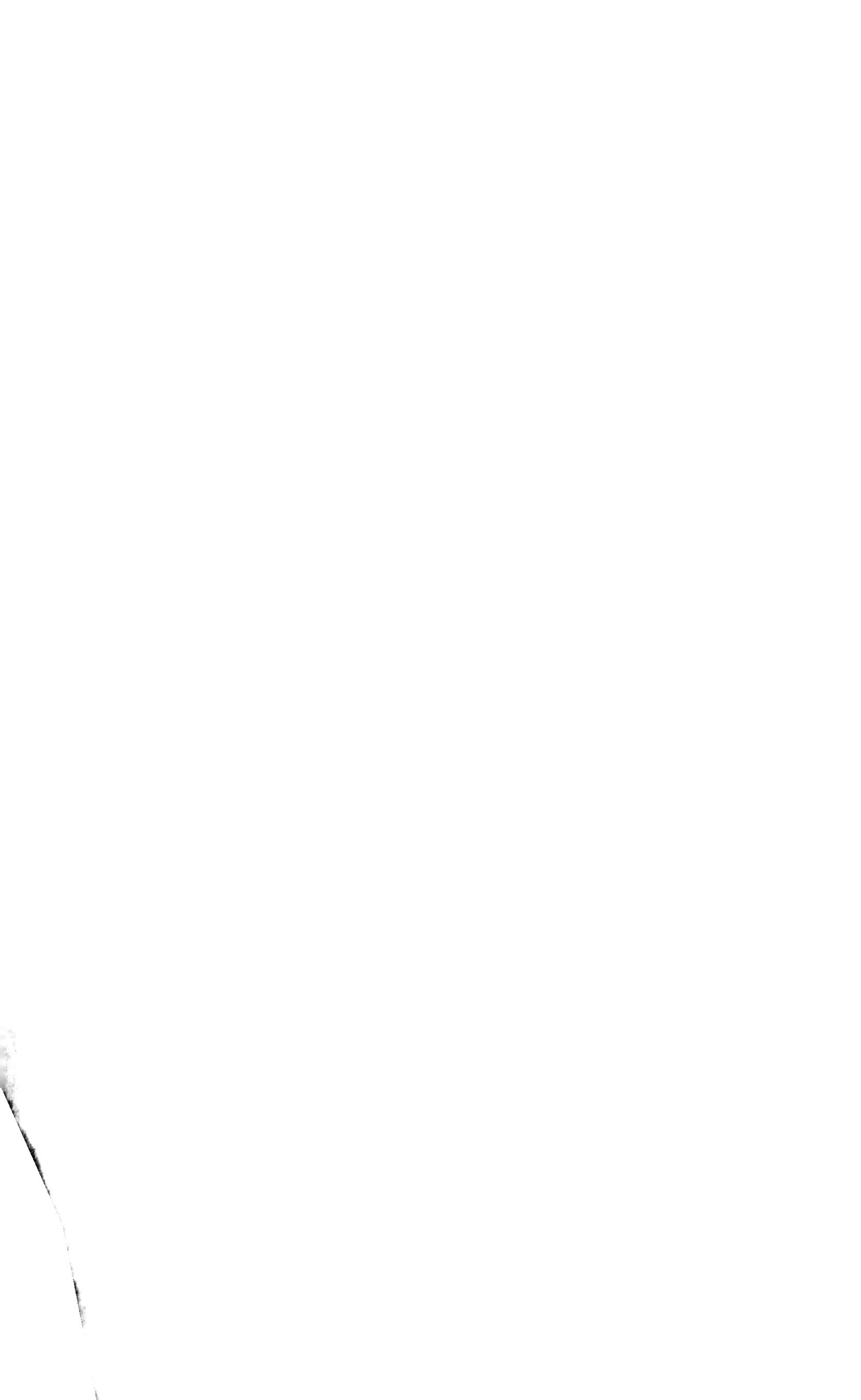